Boost Your Gut Health

"Unlocking the Power Within With Easy to Apply Measures: A Guide to Gut Health and Vitality"

Jason Higginss

Contents

Introduction

It's likely that you've heard the phrase "gut health" and that having "good" gut health is ideal. But what exactly does having a healthy stomach mean? It refers to the proper ratio of various microorganisms and microscopic bacteria in your digestive system. Researchers are learning more and more about the roles these microbes play in general health.

According to gastroenterologist Sabine Hazan, M.D., founder of Ventura Clinical Trials in Ventura, California, "having a healthy gut means you have a stronger immune system, a better mood, effective digestion that's free of discomfort and a healthy brain and heart.",

PART 1

What Does Gut Health Mean?

The state of your gastrointestinal (GI) tract, which includes digestion, a stable and normal microbiome, the absence of GI illnesses, a functioning immune system, and other factors, is referred to as gut health. Experts from Ohio State University Wexner Medical Center assert that there is a connection between the condition of your GI tract and other elements of general health, including emotional stress and chronic illness. Further evidence points to the possibility that a person's environment, habits, and diet may have an impact on their gut health.

Hormones and nerves in your stomach interact with your brain to support and preserve general health and wellbeing. A healthy gut usually has beneficial bacteria and immune cells that combat viruses and bacteria that cause disease.

Concerning Your Microbiome

According to Dr. Hazan, the microbiome is made up of all the bacteria, viruses, and fungi that live in the human body.

Skin, mouth, throat, stomach, colon, uterus, ovarian follicles, prostate, lungs, ears, and eyes are just a few of the places these bacteria can be found. Dr. Hazan asserts, "You name it, and there are microorganisms nearby," noting that studies have found that the human body has about 10,000 distinct microbial species.

Anaerobic bacteria do not require oxygen, whereas aerobic bacteria do. Microbiologists classify bacteria into these two groups. According to Dr. Hazan, bacteria that flourish in the stomach are often anaerobic, but those that dwell on the skin are aerobic. "The microbiome is crucial; it affects a wide range of illnesses, including COVID-19 and cancer."

Why Does Gut Health Matter?

Your gut, sometimes referred to as your digestive system or gastrointestinal (GI) system, breaks down the food you eat, absorbs its nutrients, and uses them to power and nourish your body.

According to Alicia Romano, a clinical dietitian at Tufts Medical Center in Boston and an official for the Academy of Nutrition and Dietetics, "the gut plays a huge role in the health and well-being of our bodies." Apart from breaking down food and taking in nutrients, the gut and brain are in close contact, regulating several aspects such as fluid secretion, GI muscle contractions, and immunological response through a continuous game of telephone.

Additionally, the gut plays a significant role in the immune system of the body—more than 70% of immune cells are found there.

Indices That Your Gut Is Not Feeling Well.

One unsettling indication that anything is wrong with your gut? Unusual alterations in your feces.

"You should be concerned if you notice sudden changes in the length, color, or consistency of your stool," advises Dr. Hazan. "Brown stool is normal; blood should never be seen in it."

Due to the fact that a large portion of the population has intestinal problems at some time in their lives, physicians created the Meyers Scale, also known as the Bristol Scale, to assist patients in describing their feces "without bringing in colored photos," according to Dr. Hazan.

Consider using the scale to help explain your worries to your doctor as various numbers correspond to different bowel movement disorders.

Nevertheless, it's critical to keep in mind what you regard as typical. Dr. Hazan explains, "If your poop has looked like Silly Putty your entire life and you don't feel any pain, this could be your normal," adding that the term "normal" is purely subjective.

There are other indications that your gut needs care in addition to the state of your bowel movements. According to Dr. Hazan, everyone should be concerned about their gut health, but certain symptoms may indicate that you should pay more attention to your gut health than others. Make an appointment with your doctor if you encounter:

unusually low body weight
Your doctor's diagnosis of anemia Pain or alteration in your bowel habits
Support for rectal bleeding A Harmonious Intestine

Using two of the probiotic strains that have been scientifically studied the most worldwide, Ritual Synbiotic+ is Made Traceable. It is intended to target bad gut bacteria, which may promote the development of good gut bacteria.

PART 2

How to Assess the Health of Your Gut

There are several ways to keep an eye on and assess your gut health if you're worried about how it's doing, both at home and with your medical professional.

Make a note of any symptoms, such as diarrhea, nausea, bloating, gas, or stomach pain. These symptoms usually go away on their own with time, but if they persist, you might need to see your doctor.

Should symptoms continue, it could be helpful to have a stool analysis performed by your medical professional. Stool analysis is a set of procedures used to examine a stool sample in order to identify and address certain gastrointestinal disorders.

Seven indicators of a sick stomach.

The gut microbiota is impacted by numerous aspects of contemporary living, such as:
excessive levels of stress, insufficient sleep, and a Western diet heavy in processed and sugary foods
using antibiotics
This could therefore have an impact on several elements of your health, like:

elevated levels of stress
inadequate sleep consuming a diet heavy in processed and sugary foods typical of the West
using antibiotics
This could therefore have an impact on several elements of your health, like:

immune system performance, hormone levels, weight, and illness development

If your gut health is compromised, you might experience a few symptoms. These are seven of the most typical indicators:

1. Distressed abdomen.

All stomach troubles may indicate a weakened digestive system. Among them are:

bloating and constipation
heartburn diarrhea

A stomach that is in balance will have an easier time breaking down food and getting rid of waste, which should result in less symptoms.

2. A diet heavy in sugar.

The diversity and quantity of "good" bacteria in your stomach can be reduced by eating a diet heavy in processed foods and added sugars.

According to research, consuming excessive amounts of sugar may cause inflammation all over the body. Numerous illnesses, including cancer, may have inflammation as a prelude. Your gut health may be harmed if you consume a lot of sugar.

3. Inadvertent fluctuations in weight.

Weight gain or loss without diet or exercise changes may indicate a gastrointestinal disorder. Your body's capacity to absorb nutrients, control blood sugar, and store fat can all be hampered by an unbalanced gut.

Malabsorption brought on by small intestine bacterial overgrowth (SIBO) may result in weight loss. Conversely, elevated inflammation or insulin resistance may be the cause of weight gain.

4. Restless nights or persistent exhaustion.

Studies suggest that sleep fragmentation and short sleep duration may be associated with an imbalance in gut flora, potentially resulting in chronic weariness.

Even if the reason is still unknownIt seems related to mental health, metabolism, and inflammation (Trusted Source).

5. Skin irritation.

The kinds of bacteria found in the stomach may be connected to skin disorders such as psoriasis. Reduced levels of good bacteria may have an effect on the health of your skin and immune system.

6. Immune disorders.

Numerous investigations have revealed links between the immune system and the stomach.

A dysfunctional digestive tract can change how well the immune system functions and raise systemic inflammation.

This could result in autoimmune illnesses, in which the body attacks itself because it believes that its own cells and organs are dangerous intruders.

7. Intolerances to food.

Food intolerances arise from problems with specific foods' digestion. This is not the same as a food allergy, which results from an adverse response of the immune system to certain foods.

Studies suggest that low-quality gut bacteria may be the source of food intolerances such as lactose intolerance. This may result in symptoms like: difficulty digesting the trigger foods

gas that bloats
nausea, vomiting, and diarrhea.
Additionally, some studies suggests a connection between intestinal health and food allergies.

PART 3

Ten Research-Proven Strategies to Boost Your Gut Health

Your gut health can be naturally improved by eating certain foods and adopting healthy lifestyle practices.

1. Consume Foods Packed with Probiotics and Fiber.

According to study, fiber, a nutrient derived from plants, lowers the risk of metabolic illnesses by promoting the diversity and proliferation of beneficial bacteria in the gut. Beets, carrots, fennel, sweet potatoes, and spinach are natural sources of fiber that improves the gut flora. Whole grains are a great source of fiber in addition to fruits and vegetables.

Because they include probiotics, fermented foods like yogurt, kimchi, sauerkraut, and kombucha are also highly valued for their capacity to strengthen the gut. Particularly, yogurt may relieve gastrointestinal ailments such constipation, diarrhea, and inflammatory bowel disease.

According to one study, those who regularly consume yogurt have lower levels of enterobacterium, a type of bacteria linked to inflammation, and higher levels of lactobacilli, a gut-beneficial bacteria, in their intestines.

2. Work Out Frequently.

For the microbiota among many other elements of the human body, movement is medication. Researchers have discovered that exercise encourages an increase in the diversity of beneficial bacteria in the gut in both human and animal experiments.

While a number of studies demonstrate the beneficial effects that food and exercise can have on gut health, a 2019 study found that exercise alone has the ability to change the composition and functionality of gut bacteria.

In terms of overall wellness, the researchers discovered that lengthier sessions and high-intensity aerobic training in particular contributed most to the diversity and function of gut flora. They also found that slim persons are more likely than overweight or obese people to benefit from exercise's benefits for gut health.

3. Restrict Your Consumption of Alcohol.

Excessive drinking can also have a harmful impact on your microbiome. Frequent alcohol use has been connected to gastritis, an inflammatory digestive condition.

Inflammation of this kind can result in bacterial infections, ulcers, persistent pain, and heartburn.

Excessive drinking is also linked to intestinal inflammation, a symptom of a malfunctioning digestive system. According to research, this type of inflammation can upset the microbiota's equilibrium and change how well it functions.

4. Lower Stress Intensities.

Consider the butterflies you get when you're nervous or excited. Stress isn't only mental. Gut health experts frequently mention the "gut-brain connection" and call the gut "the second brain." Even though we don't fully understand their relationship, we do know that there is a close connection between gut health and mental health.

According to research, the stomach influences anxiety and depression and vice versa; these mental health conditions can raise the risk of IBS, and those who have IBS are more likely to suffer from these mental health conditions.

Reducing painful GI symptoms and restoring balance to your body may be possible by learning how to manage your stress and mental health. Not sure where to begin? Consider including some exercise in your daily routine.

A daily stroll could have a positive impact on gut health because, according to study, exercise can enhance the number and quality of gut microorganisms that promote health.

5. Take Into Account an Addendum.

The popularity of probiotic supplements has grown as awareness of the significance of gut health has risen. Although probiotic supplements aren't a cure-all for gut health, there is some evidence that, in some circumstances, they help strengthen the microbiota and improve gut health.

Probiotics may help with a number of health issues, including reducing the risk of infections when taking antibiotics and reducing inflammation in those with inflammatory bowel disease who also suffer from pouchitis. But not every health issue is a good fit for every probiotic, and the majority of probiotics are probably
restricted in their potential to improve gut health, particularly in the absence of other beneficial decisions.

Speak with your physician if probiotic supplements pique your curiosity. Even though these supplements are generally thought to be safe, particularly for healthy individuals, those with weakened immune systems are more susceptible to negative consequences.

6. Get adequate rest.

Your gut health may suffer significantly if you don't get enough or high-quality sleep, and this might exacerbate your sleep problems.

Make it a priority to obtain 7–8 hours of unbroken sleep every night from a reliable source. If you have problems falling asleep, your doctor might be able to assist.

7. Consume food gradually.

Eating more slowly and properly chewing your food will help you make healthier food choices and reduce your risk of obesity and diabetes.

By doing this, you might be able to lessen gastrointestinal pain and preserve gut health.

8. Continue to drink water.

Although the source of the water is important, drinking a lot of water may be associated with a greater diversity of bacteria in the stomach.

Additionally, a 2022 study discovered that a certain type of bacteria linked to gastrointestinal diseases was less common in those who drank more water.

Constipation can be avoided and general health advantages can be obtained from drinking enough water. It can also be an easy method to support intestinal health.

9. Examine any dietary intolerances.

If you have symptoms like bloating or abdominal pain, you might have a food intolerance.

gas and diarrhea

emesis weariness acid reflux

To test whether your symptoms get better, you can try avoiding foods that are frequently triggers. It's possible that your digestive health will improve if you can recognize and stay away from the food or items causing your symptoms.

10. Modify your food intake.

You may improve your gut health by consuming fewer processed, sugary, and high-fat foods.

A healthy gut flora is probably also influenced by eating a diet rich in fiber. Eating foods high in polyphenols, which are micronutrients found in foods,

Fruits, veggies, coffee, tea, and alcohol

Four dietary categories for intestinal health

Gut health and diet seem to be closely related. Since these foods may encourage the growth of harmful bacteria, avoiding processed meals, high-fat foods, and foods high in refined sugars is probably vital for keeping a healthy microbiome.

Certain meals can actively encourage the growth of good bacteria in your body, improving your general health. The following are some superfoods for intestinal health:

1. Diets high in fiber.

Foods rich in fiber appear to benefit gut health, according to research. Among these foods are:

entire grains, such as quinoa and oats; legumes, such as black beans and chickpeas; vegetables, such as broccoli and asparagus; nuts, such as almonds and pistachios; fruits, such as apples and peaches.

2. Onion

Garlic may boost gut microbiota diversity and enhance gut health, per a 2019 rodent study.

In a similar vein, a small 2018 study including 49 participants discovered that aged garlic extract raised the diversity and quantity of good bacteria. However, more human study ought to be conducted.

3. Foods that have undergone fermentation.

Good sources of probiotics for the diet are fermented foods. Some examples are yogurt kefir, sauerkraut, and kimchi.

Consuming these meals may enhance gut microbiome, according to research.

4. Foods that increase collagen.

Foods high in collagen, such salmon skin and bone broth, may be good for your intestinal health as well as your general health.

Collagen supplementation may improve the gut ecology in mice, according to a 2021 study, although more investigation is required.

You may also attempt to increase the amount of collagen your body produces by eating differently. To enhance your body's collagen production, try consuming more:

Broccoli, meat, eggs, orange fruits, and nuts.

Why do people's gut microbiota compositions differ from one another?

The gut microbiota is influenced by numerous factors, including:

antibiotic use, diet, genetics, environment, stress, and sleep

Each of these elements varies from person to person and affects gut microbiomes in a unique way. This variance leads to differences in the gut microbiomes of individuals.

What effect does fasting have on the gut microbiome? Research on humans is still lacking, but fasting appears to benefit the gut microbiome, as evidenced by a small 2019 study involving 16 participants that found a connection between fasting and lower levels of a bacteria linked to colorectal cancer. Research on animals also demonstrates the benefits of fasting, with one study in 2018 finding that intermittent fasting appeared to improve gut health and increase lifespan, and another in 2019 finding that fasting promoted the growth of beneficial gut bacteria and reduced inflammation in the intestines.

Can the gut microbiome be altered by consuming probiotics?

According to certain research, probiotics have no effect on the gut microbiota. Nevertheless, several studies indicate that probiotics could have a major impact on the composition of the gut microbiome and enhance other aspects of health, such as immunity.

How can I strengthen the health of my gut?

Making improvements to your general health can help your gut health. This can involve consuming a diet higher in fiber, consuming fewer highly processed foods, obtaining adequate sleep, and controlling your stress levels.

What symptoms indicate gut health issues?
Fatigue, inadvertent weight changes, and unsettled stomach are a few symptoms of an imbalanced gut flora.

The human digestive system is intricate. Even though studies are still being conducted, it appears that the gut microbiota has an effect on overall health. A healthy digestive system supports:

a robust defense mechanism

heart health, brain health, mood enhancement, sound sleep, efficient digestion, and possible protection against certain malignancies and autoimmune illnesses

A change in diet and lifestyle may have a favorable impact on your general health as well as the health of your gut.

A change in diet and lifestyle may have a favorable impact on your general health as well as the health of your gut.

Summary

A trip to the doctor may be helpful if you have symptoms like blood in your stool, unexplained stomach pain, unusual weight loss, or altered bowel habits. For the purpose of diagnosing, treating, or ruling out specific medical diseases, your doctor might order a number of tests.

www.ingramcontent.com/pod-product-compliance
Lightning Source LLC
Chambersburg PA
CBHW070752260726
48660CB00007B/3079